A Yogi's Guide to

Chakra Meditation

Paul Grilley

Acknowledgements:

Thank you Stephanie Hii for your illustrations.

Thank you Joe Barnett for copy editing, and editing, and editing…

Thank you my friends for your encouragement and your help in making this publication possible:

Murielle Burellier
Bernie Clark
Anat Geiger
Jo Phee
Sebastian Pucelle
Paul Terrell
Marcel van de Vis Heil

Printed in the United States of America

ISBN 978-1-7335839-0-9

PaulGrilleyAuthor@gmail.com

To Suzee.

Thousands of walks,

thousands of talks,

thousands of hours of practice,

you helped form and refine all I have written.

TABLE OF CONTENTS

FOREWORD

The most respected text in the yogic tradition was written by the sage Patanjali and is entitled "The Yoga Sutras." Scholars debate its antiquity, but it was written approximately 2000 years ago. Because an overview of Patanjali's Yoga Sutras is standard fare in yoga teacher training programs, I have presented chakra meditation as a specific example of Patanjali's more general description of yoga. I hope that a description of chakra meditation through Patanjali's lens will make it easier for yoginis coming to this material for the first time. I have included references to Patanjali's sutras at the appropriate places.

My spiritual teacher was Dr. Hiroshi Motoyama. He passed from this earth September 19, 2015. Because he wrote in so many fields of study, it is difficult to summarize his teachings succinctly, but central to them was his scientific attitude toward all things, including spiritual practices.

The scientific attitude is test, test, test, then change a variable, and test again.

I have suggested several techniques in this manual. My suggestions are based on years of studying and practicing yoga. But I know from discussions with students and colleagues that no person responds to any suggested technique or routine in exactly the same way. Each student must modify each technique in a way best suited to his or her unique physiology and psychology. This attitude is fundamental to Dr. Motoyama's approach to yoga practice. He constantly suggested variations of the pranayama and meditation techniques that he taught. And he frequently ended his lectures with this advice:

"You must proceed with the courage and self-confidence to test these things for yourself."

Paul Grilley,
Watsonville, CA
February 2019

PART 1.
CHAKRA THEORY.

Seven chakras. Modern people unquestioningly accept the premise that consciousness is centered in the brain. But tantric texts describe seven primary centers of consciousness, two of which are in the brain and five more in the spinal cord. These seven centers of consciousness are called "chakras," and within these chakras are the seeds of our karma.

There are technical manuals in tantric literature that describe more than seven chakras, but these additional chakras can be considered aspects or polarities of the seven chakras. It is my premise that when the seven primary chakras awaken, all the related or subsidiary chakras also awaken.

Sushumna. All seven chakras are part of a central channel of energy called "sushumna." Sushumna runs from your coccyx, up your spine, and extends out beyond the top of your head.

In the physical body, sushumna is related to the cerebral spinal fluid that surrounds and penetrates the brain and spinal cord.

Brahman's Gate. The place where sushumna pierces the top of your head can be felt as a shallow indentation where bones of the skull knit together. This shallow indentation is called a fontanel in modern anatomy. It is called "Brahman's Gate" in yogic literature.

Location of the chakras. Each chakra has a "root" area and a "flower" area. The root of a chakra is in the spine. The flower of a chakra spreads out from the root and disperses over a larger area. When practicing chakra meditation, yoginis concentrate on the root or the flower of a chakra, or they imagine a sphere of energy that includes both the root and the flower of a chakra.

NAME	ROOT LOCATION	FLOWER LOCATION
7. Sahasrara	Upper Brain	Brahman's Gate
6. Ajna	Brain Center	Third Eye
5. Vishuddha	7th Cervical Vertebra	Throat
4. Anahata	5th Thoracic Vertebra	Heart
3. Manipura	2nd Lumbar Vertebra	Upper Abdomen
2. Svadhisthana	2nd Sacral Vertebra	Lower Abdomen
1. Muladhara	Coccyx	Pelvic Floor

Subjective locations. Don't be anxious about exactly locating a chakra's physical position. When practicing yoga, your subjective experience of a chakra is most important. For example, ajna chakra is described as being in the center of the brain, but in my experience it is slightly behind and below the center of my brain.

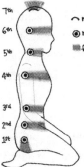

root location of Sahasrara
root location of chakras
flower location of chakras

ROOT AND FLOWER OF CHAKRAS

Shiva and Shakti. In the beginning, there was no universe. There was only the Unmanifested Absolute. Then the Absolute manifested two interacting poles: Consciousness and Energy. Tantric yogis call these two poles "Shiva and Shakti." Shiva is the conscious witness of all things in the universe. Shakti is the power that manifests all the changing things that Shiva witnesses. This is the Fundamental Dualism.

Not two. The Fundamental Dualism is not absolute; Shiva influences Shakti, and Shakti influences Shiva. Shiva is not a powerless witness; Shiva has the power of intention. Shiva's intentions influence what Shakti manifests. Shakti is not a bundle of inanimate energies; Shakti is also conscious. Shakti consciously responds to the intentions of Shiva. Dr. Motoyama believed the Taoist Taijitu symbol (see next page) to be the best artistic expression of how Shiva and Shakti are two aspects of the same Reality that mutually influence each other.

Shiva-prana and Shakti-prana. Every human being is a blend of a small portion of Shiva and Shakti. The breadth, clarity, and depth of your awareness constitute your portion of Shiva's power, your "Shiva-prana." Your body, physical sensations, sensory perceptions, emotions, thoughts, and memories constitute your portion of Shakti's power, your "Shakti-prana." These pranas, these powers, are constantly influencing each other.

Mutual influence. When a yogini sits to meditate, her Shiva-prana, her awareness, becomes aware of her Shakti-prana, her sensations, memories, emotions, and thoughts. If she doesn't exercise her power of intention, then her thoughts "run all over the place," or she will not be able to "get a thought out of her head." These are examples of Shakti-prana influencing Shiva-prana. But a meditating yogini can use her power of intention, her will, to visualize a chakra, or recover a memory, or follow a line of reasoning. These are examples of her Shiva-prana influencing the manifestations of Shakti-prana.

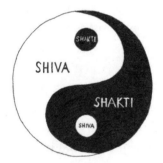

RELATION OF SHIVA-PRANA TO SHAKTI-PRANA

Four dimensions of existence. The Unmanifested Absolute manifests as Shiva and Shakti. The first manifestation of Shiva and Shakti is what Dr. Motoyama called "The Realm of Purusha." From the realm of Purusha, three other realms, or dimensions of existence, are created. They are the causal, the astral, and the physical.

Purusha. The ancients referred to this dimension as the world of the gods. Purushas are not limited by bodies. Their consciousness can expand to include a mountain, or a planet, or a galaxy, or all of creation. Or their consciousness can shrink to the size of a microbe. The birth or death of a body is experienced without any interruption in their awareness. Your true nature is to exist as an immortal Purusha. (Patanjali 1.3, 4.34)

Causal, astral, physical. From a part of the realm of Purusha, the causal dimension is created. It is the realm of thought and ideas. From a part of the causal dimension, the astral dimension is created. It is the realm of emotion and desire. And from a part of the astral dimension, the physical dimension is created.

A body is a boundary. Each of the four dimensions is populated with created beings, and each being has a body suitable for that dimension. A body marks a boundary between what is you and what is not you. If you are a physically embodied being, then you live in a state of tension with your physical environment. You need your environment; you cannot exist without it. You need to take from your environment all the food, water, air, and other things you need to exist. But there are aspects of your environment that are a constant threat to your existence. Too much heat or cold, too little food or water, or a tiger, or a bacteria: all of these things could end your physical existence. Your needs are endless and so are the threats. Hope and fear are the inevitable consequences of being embodied.

Three bodies. A causal being has a causal body. An astral being has a causal and an astral body. A physical being has a causal, an astral, and a physical body. Human beings are ensheathed by three bodies. (Patanjali 3.38, 3.43-3.50)

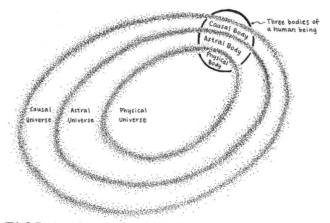

THREE WORLDS AND THREE BODIES

The causal body. The causal dimension is sometimes called the "Realm of Ideas." Your thoughts and beliefs make up your causal body. But these ideas are not merely factual things like "Paris is the capital of France." They are your beliefs of what is right, what is true, and what is good. Causal ideas create your personality: they are your view of life and the world. These beliefs are such a basic foundation of our personalities that we rarely question their existence or clearly articulate what they are.

Your causal body is composed of your opinions and beliefs about life: Is there a soul? Is there a God? Is there karma or justice? Is there life after death? How big is the universe? Are all races of men equal? Are men and women equal? Is there such a thing as free will?

The paradox of your causal body of beliefs is that they have the strongest influence over your behavior, yet you are generally unaware of what they are until your world view is confronted by someone else's. Hence the old saying: "Do not talk about politics or religion at the dinner table."

We are more attached to our causal bodies of belief than to our physical bodies. People are willing to kill themselves or others for their beliefs. Spiritually immature people find any confrontation with their beliefs too painful to endure. Insisting that one's own ideas are absolutely correct becomes religious or political fundamentalism.

A spiritually mature person contemplates why she believes what she believes and why she reacts in the ways that she does. Experience has taught her that many of her beliefs were wrong or inadequate. Examining one's own beliefs requires empathy, honesty, and sometimes painful self-assessments.

The astral body. The English language is quite lax when it comes to distinguishing between causal and astral "feelings." Causal feelings are centered on impersonal ideas such as patriotism, religious beliefs, or social justice. Certainly, we "feel" strongly about these ideas. We might willingly die for them. But they are impersonal in nature. Astral feelings are more accurately considered "emotions" that are centered on personal concerns such as health, wealth, romance, and reputation. Your personal desires form your astral body.

The astral dimension is sometimes called the "Realm of Form and Desire." It is the realm where you create the plans and gather the energy for your personal fulfillment, your personal hopes and desires. The defining characteristic of astral thinking is creating a narrative of your own life in which you are the star. Causal thoughts are about the nature of the world or society. But astral thoughts are about "Me." What do I want? What is my passion? How can I succeed?

Historical narratives can be boring if we don't identify with any particular character. Novelists make history "come alive" by telling a story through the hopes and fears of a character. In this way, we become "emotionally invested" in the story. Such emotions are of the astral realm.

Astral thinking is colored by "like and dislike" because it has a strong preference for "Me." Selfish people put personal welfare before duty. Virtuous people do the opposite. If a captain abandoned his post while his ship was sinking, he would be despised. Overcoming emotional, selfish thinking is an essential discipline to gain control over your astral body.

People who patiently cultivate the ability to think and act without personal preference are rightly admired, whether they be ship captains, parents, judges, or counselors. There is no benefit in degrading yourself or thinking yourself less than another. But to gain control over your astral body, you must be guided by something higher than your egoistic concerns.

The physical body. The physical dimension is the world you experience through your physical body and physical senses. It is the "real world" of the materialist. In the physical dimension, you feel that your thoughts and emotions are separate from the outer world of the senses, but in the astral world, this is not the case. In the astral world, animals, plants, and even the weather are influenced by your thoughts and emotions. In the astral world, a soul with a strong will can alter the form of the food that it eats, such as altering an apple into a pear. Thoughts and emotions also affect objects in the physical world. But this influence is usually so small that scientists tend to deny such things. Most people could stare at an apple all day, and there would be no noticeable change.

Dr. Motoyama said that a newborn baby still has astral awareness; she still sees and reacts to beings in the astral world. This is why she only sometimes focuses her physical eyes on physical objects. The physical world seems the most real to us now because we no longer directly perceive beings of the astral or causal worlds.

Chakras convert energy. The three bodies constantly interact with each other. The energies of causal ideas are converted into astral emotions and desires. The energies of astral emotions and desires are converted into physical sensations and actions. Each of these energy conversions occurs in the chakras. The three bodies are knit together at the chakras.

What is fundamental to chakra theory is that energy conversions occur in both directions. The process of embodiment is a conversion of energies from causal to astral to physical manifestations. The process of disembodiment is a conversion of energies in the opposite direction: from physical to astral to causal.

Chakra meditation. A yogini begins by concentrating physical energies into a chakra. This increases the physical sensations of heat, pressure, and vibration. If a yogini continues to concentrate on the chakra, it will awaken and convert the physical energies into astral manifestations of light, images, memory, and desire. If the yogini remains unmoved by these astral energies and continues to concentrate on the chakra, then the chakra will awaken to an even higher level of function and convert astral energies into causal manifestations of insight and understanding. In this way, chakra meditation ascends upward from physical sensations, to astral emotions, to causal ideas, and finally, freedom from the limitations of all three bodies, the realm of Purusha.

The conversion of energies is not always in a linear, causal-astral-physical sequence. Causal energies can convert directly into physical manifestations, and physical energies can convert directly into causal manifestations. Physical exercise can relieve causal preoccupations. A change in your causal beliefs can energize and even heal your physical body. This is why your "sadhana," your spiritual practices should include physical exercise and philosophical study.

Worlds of Karma. Dr. Motoyama called the causal, astral, and physical dimensions "The Worlds of Karma." Every action you perform in these dimensions has an equal and balancing reaction. You will continue to be reborn in these dimensions until the karmic scales have balanced.

In the physical dimension, if you push an object, the object pushes back with equal force. In the astral dimension, your courtesy and kindness are rewarded. But if you bully or ostracize someone, you will suffer the same. In the causal dimension, if you refuse to examine your beliefs or if you are dishonest, then you will become unable to think clearly.

Karma and desire. Two types of forces draw you into rebirth: "karmic debts" and unsatisfied desires. The length of time between your actions and their karmic reactions varies. Sometimes, instant karma does get you. But at other times, it can be years or even lifetimes before the karma-balancing reaction occurs. Karmic debts are those reactions to your actions that have not yet manifested.

Even if you have no karmic debts, if you cling to your desires, you will be drawn into new births. You will reincarnate again and again until you have satisfied your desires or you have released them. And each time you reincarnate, you will be tempted to form new desires.

Karmic seeds. All of your karmic debts and unsatisfied desires lie dormant as seeds in your chakras. They will awaken in future lives when social circumstances allow them to sprout and seek fulfillment. (Patanjali 3.18-3.20, 4.2-4.11)

Wheel of Samsara. Your causal, astral, and physical bodies are formed and maintained by the chakras. The strengths and weaknesses of each body are determined by which kinds of karmic seeds are active in each of the chakras.

All bodies are created things. All created things perish. Embodied souls suffer because they seek immortality and unending happiness in a physical world of constant change, decay, and death. Fear of suffering or death leads to selfish choices which create more karma. This cycle of desire, karma-creating actions, death, and reincarnation is called the "Wheel of Samsara."

Abiding as Purusha. But when a soul knows itself as Purusha, as unembodied consciousness, then the terrors and disappointments of embodied existence end. The soul continues to act, but it acts with wisdom so that it doesn't create new karma. Such a soul effectively settles its karmic debts and can be a great help to others because it acts so selflessly.

Enlightened yoginis are neither inert nor removed from the endless drama of creation, but they are free of the delusion that they are the bodies through which the drama of creation is experienced. Bodies come and go, but our true nature, consciousness, is beyond the reach of birth, growth, decay, and death.

The goal of chakra meditation is to slowly and systematically untangle the karmic threads that bind your consciousness to your physical, astral, and causal bodies and to reach again the free world of Purusha, disembodied existence. Only then will you be "abiding in your own true nature." (Patanjali 1.3, 4.34)

Part 2.
Yoga Theory.

Translating chakra theory into yoga theory. "Tantra" means "system" or "scientific theory" or "magical formula." Tantric texts are usually written as dialogues that expound the theory of creation. They also describe techniques and rituals that lead to spiritual powers or spiritual liberation. Tantra claims great antiquity for its tradition, but the texts known to us are about 1500 years old. Shiva, Shakti, and chakras are conceptions that are central to tantric texts, but since most yoga practicitoners are more familiar with Patanjali's Yoga Sutras, I wish to use his terms for describing the practice of meditation.

Patanjali's word for Universal Consciousness isn't Shiva; it is *Purusha*.

Patanjali's word for Universal Energy isn't Shakti; it is *Prakriti*.

Patanjali's word for each human being's experience of Shiva isn't Shiva-prana; it is *chitta*.

Patanjali's word for each human being's experience of Shakti isn't Shakti-prana; it is *vritti*.

In Patanjali's system, the yogini's essential nature is Purusha, but she is not "abiding" in this nature. She is not aware of all things in the universe. She is only aware of the vrittis in her chitta. The goal of yoga is to slowly expand a yogini's awareness until she is no longer limited to her chitta, but is one with that special Purusha which is omniscient and untouched by suffering. (Patanjali 1.2-1.4, 1.23-1.28, 2.45, 4.34)

Patanjali defines yoga this way:

Yoga is the control of the vrittis in the chitta.
(Patanjali 1.2)

Chitta. In yoga theory your individual field of awareness is called "chitta," and anything you are aware of is called a "vritti." All your thoughts, memories, emotions, physical sensations, and sensory perceptions are called vrittis. A modern English speaker would say, "I have something on my mind." Patanjali would say, "I have a vritti in my chitta."

Physical vrittis. These are what first beset the beginner in meditation. They include physical restlessness, fatigue, and sensitivity to heat, or cold, or noise. The yogini must become indifferent to physical and sensory stimuli.

Astral vrittis. These are emotions and desires. They reflect your frustrations and infatuations. They include memories of success and failure, strong emotions, and unfulfilled ambitions.

Causal vrittis. These are deep questions that are usually brought up by some distress or disappointment. Why did that happen? Why is the world the way it is? What is the purpose of life?

Controlling the vrittis. If your chitta is like the surface of a pond, then your vrittis are like waves on that surface. As soon as one wave dies away, countless other physical, emotional, and intellectual stimuli give rise to new waves of vrittis. The new wave could be a bodily sensation such as thirst, or a sensory perception such as a noise, or a memory that arises, or an inspiring insight about your life. Some waves might flit by almost unnoticed, but others might start a long chain of related thoughts, feelings, and memories. Yogananda wrote that the average person has thousands of "thoughts" in a day. Controlling these thoughts, these vrittis, is yoga.

Beneath your awareness. A thought can be present but not noticed. A mundane example is when you hum a song to yourself but are unaware of it until your roommate asks you to stop. More consequential examples include dark musings of resentment against your boss or uplifting thoughts of devotion. Habits of thought are important because they create a mental background that is subliminally influencing your behavior. You want this background to be uplifting, not negative or depressing.

Vasanas and samskaras. The seeds of all your habits of behavior and unsatisfied desires are stored in the appropriate chakras. When a desire is dormant or beneath your awareness, it is called a "vasana." When a habit is dormant or beneath your awareness, it is called a "samskara." When you become aware of a desire, or a habit, or a thought, they are called vrittis.

Chakra purification. When you concentrate your energy and awareness on a chakra, you inevitably energize and awaken the vasanas and samskaras stored there. This phase of spiritual development is called chakra purification. Newly awakened vasanas of desire and samskaras of behavior have much more power than the active vrittis of your everyday mundane preoccupations. They include all the unfinished goals, dreams, frustrations, and disappointments that you have accumulated. The deeper the vasana, the stronger it is. Facing them and dissolving them are necessary aspects of spiritual growth.

Danger of chakra purification. When long suppressed vasanas awaken, you might start to question many of your life choices: your marriage, your job, your goals. You might be tempted to blame your family and friends for the irritating duties and restrictions of your present life. This is a huge mistake. It is easy to be seduced into pursuing newly awakened desires and to forget that the arising of strong desires is just an aspect of chakra purification.

Afflicted vrittis. Patanjali didn't use the term "chakra purification." He used the term "afflicted vrittis." They are afflicted because they must be resolved before a meditator can advance. (Patanjali 1.4-1.5)

Patanjali outlined a three-pronged strategy for resolving afflicted vrittis.

1. **Dismiss them.** Some vrittis are just distracting, mundane concerns; they should be dismissed. (Patanjali 1.12-1.16)

2. **Neutralize them.** Mentally rehearse the opposite quality. For example, if you cannot stop thinking about someone's rudeness, then mentally rehearse forgiving him. (Patanjali 2.33-2.34)

3. **Retrace them.** Some vrittis are deep and emotionally charged. They should be examined and dissolved. Concerns about health, or work, or relationships are common vrittis which are difficult to dismiss. Patanjali suggests retracing these vrittis back to their origin: When and why did they originate? Why did you get involved? What did you expect to gain from these relationships? This is an effective way to gain insight into your preoccupations and attachments. (Patanjali 2.3-2.10, 4.23-4.28)

Empty nests. When a memory, or habit, or desire has become so weak that it can be put aside and not disturb your meditation, then you have purified that vritti. These memories and desires still exist, but they no longer have power to compel you to do things detrimental to your spiritual progress. Dr. Motoyama referred to such powerless vrittis as "empty nests."

Nonafflicted vrittis. Patanjali defined two broad categories of vrittis: "afflicted" and "nonafflicted." Both forms of vrittis must be resolved but not in the same way. Afflicted vrittis should be "dismissed," "neutralized," or "retraced." Nonafflicted vrittis should be cultivated because they "calm and clarify the mind." (Patanjali 1.33-1.40)

There are numerous forms of nonafflicted vrittis, and it would be impossible to list them all. They include uplifting feelings of peace, of love, calm insights into your own behavior, pleasant memories of kindness, or an inner reconciliation with those who have passed beyond this world. You should allow yourself to become absorbed into them and absorb strength from them. They will eventually fade, and then you should lovingly set them aside and return to your focus on the chakras.

Chakra awakening. Nonafflicted vrittis, such as memories and insights into your history and behavior, are important. But they still belong to the phase of spiritual development that Dr. Motoyama called chakra purification. This means they are related to your own past actions, good and bad. As you pass beyond chakra purification, you enter the phase of spiritual development that Dr. Motoyama called chakra awakening. When a chakra begins to awaken, some of the vrittis that arise will not be the result of your present day preoccupations or past actions. They will be the direct perception of the astral or causal worlds, and the beings that inhabit them. (Patanjali 3.23-3.55)

Special vrittis. In chakra meditation, there are three types of nonafflicted vrittis that are particularly beneficial. They will take you into deeper meditations. They are energy movement, astral lights, and "nada sounds."

1. **Energy movement**. This is experienced as sensations of pressure or vibration or heat. Frequently, these sensations are not limited to a single chakra but spread throughout sushumna or other parts of the body. Tantric texts have detailed many different ways Shakti-prana can move within sushumna: crawling along your spine like ants, or hopping like a frog from one chakra to the next, or undulating along your spine like a serpent. I do not list all of them here but encourage you to pay attention to all the subtle changes of energy movement that occur within you.

2. **Astral lights.** Chakras radiate astral lights which can be seen reflected in the third eye, the flower of the sixth chakra. Try to be sensitive to every subtle shift of the shimmering light that occurs at your third eye. (Patanjali 2.52, 3.32)

3. **Nada sounds.** Chakras vibrate with astral sounds. These sounds are called nada. The nada of the first chakra is said to be like a buzzing bee; the second chakra is like a flute; the third is like a harp; the

fourth is like a large bell; the fifth is like ocean waves; and the sixth and seventh are the harmonious combination of all these sounds as OM. Of course, these descriptions are approximate.

In the beginning, the nada sounds are heard in your right ear, but with time, they are heard in both ears and centered in the back of your head. Try to become absorbed into whatever nada sounds you hear. You might hear several sounds at once, or one sound might dominate.

OM is the primordial vibration that creates and sustains the universe. The nada sounds emanating from each of the chakras are just partial refractions of OM. The true OM, the complete OM contains all sounds in it and is reverberating everywhere in the universe. Yogananda wrote that if you meditate on nada sounds, you will eventually be drawn upward into a perception of the primordial OM vibration. (Patanjali 1.23-1.29)

Part 3.
Eight Limbs of Yoga.

Eight limbs of yoga. Patanjali organized all variety of yogic practices into eight limbs. Each of the eight limbs is a form of controlling the vrittis in your chitta. They begin with the crudest techniques for controlling your outward behavior and end with the subtlest techniques for controlling your mind. (Patanjali 2.29)

1. **Yama.** Control your interactions with others.
   Don't hurt people. Don't steal. Tell the truth. Don't be greedy. Control your sexual impulses.

2. **Niyama**. Control your personal habits of behavior.
   Practice cleanliness. Practice calmness. Practice self-discipline. Practice rituals that stir your devotion. Meditate on OM.

3. **Asana**. Sit with an upright spine, in a stable and comfortable posture.
   Sit still to gain control over your impulses to move.

4. **Pranayama**. Control your prana.
   Learn to move your internal energy by controlling your breathing.

5. **Pratyahara.** Withdraw energy from the sensory nerves.
   Draw the energy away from your senses and into sushumna. This shields the mind from external distractions.

6. **Dharana**. Concentrate on the physical location of a chakra. This is usually combined with pranayama or a mantra.

7. **Dhyana**. Meditate on an inner experience.
   Become absorbed into the subtle phenomena that arise, such as energy movement or nada sounds.

8. **Samadhi**. A change in identity.
   Free yourself from any attachment to your physical body of sensations, or your astral body of emotions and desires, or your causal body of beliefs. Patanjali says that if you succeed, then you will be "abiding in your own true nature." (Patanjali 1.3)

Yama and niyama. Yama and niyama are the first two limbs of yogic control. Controlling your behavior is the first step toward controlling the vrittis in your chitta. This is why Patanjali lists basic tenets of social and personal behavior as the first two of his eight limbs of yoga. Yamas have to do with social behaviors. Niyamas have to do with personal habits.

Each of the first five chakras is host to particular types of afflicted vrittis. Listed below are the dominant vrittis, and the yamas and niyamas that neutralize them. (Patanjali 2.30-2.45)

5th Chakra

Afflicted vrittis: Pride of family, caste, race, or social status.

Yama: Satya. Be truthful, examine your motivations.

Niyama: Ishvara-pranidhana. Meditate on OM and contemplate its significance.

4th Chakra

Afflicted vrittis: Aggression, the desire to control the behavior of others.

Yama: Ahimsa. Do not be jealous or desire people to suffer for their faults.

Niyama: Santosha. Practice contentment and gratitude.

3rd Chakra

Afflicted vrittis: Constantly complaining, easily annoyed.

Yama: Aparigraha. Simplify your life, luxury wastes time and money.

Niyama: Tapas. Be patient, discipline your body and mind.

2nd Chakra

Afflicted vrittis: Sexual obsession.

Yama: Brahmacharya. Do not let sex compromise your work or relationships.

Niyama: Svadhyaya. Raise your ideals through spiritual studies and practices.

1st Chakra

Afflicted vrittis: Desire for sensory experience, attachment to the body.

Yama: Asteya. Do not steal.

Niyama: Shaucha. Keep your body clean.

Asana. Asana is the third limb of yogic control. Patanjali defines asana as "a steady and comfortable posture." Sitting upright and still for long periods of time is a difficult practice, not just physically but also mentally. Sitting in stillness reveals the intimate connection between mind and body. Sitting in stillness reveals your mental processes by inhibiting their physical expression. (Patanjali 2.46-2.48)

Every vritti of sensation, emotion, and thought affects your body. Physical sensations of heat, or cold, or discomfort prompt you to shift your sitting position, or scratch, or cough. Astral memories and emotions also create impulses to move. And even if these impulses are suppressed, these astral vrittis cause involuntary changes to your breathing rate, heart rate, blood pressure, eye movements, and nervous sensitivity. Causal memories and thoughts also affect your astral emotions and physical movements.

Most of us would be shocked to see how our facial expressions and body movements are constantly changing to reflect the vrittis in our chittas. A film of the average person's day would reveal hundreds of unconscious facial expressions, eye movements, head movements, hand gestures, and physical posturing. Poker players and police interrogators use these signs in their professions. Sitting in stillness makes us aware of these vrittis. It is a common misconception for a beginning meditator to say, "I don't like to sit. It makes my mind too busy!" Actually this meditator is becoming aware of how busy her mind always is.

A yogini need not sit cross-legged; any position in which she can comfortably hold her spine upright is adequate, even sitting in a chair. But it is important not to slump forward or lean backward against a support. Holding yourself upright develops your will, keeps you alert, and helps ensure the free flow of energy within sushumna.

Pranayama. Pranayama is the fourth limb of yogic control. Pranayama is a compound of two words prana + yama. Prana means life energy; yama means control. Pranayama is learning to control the movement of energy in your body. In chakra meditation, pranayama is the ability to move Shiva-prana and Shakti-prana up and down sushumna. Patanjali defines pranayama as "controlling the ingoing and outgoing breaths." (Patanjali 2.49-2.51)

Shiva-prana. Your consciousness, your Shiva-prana is everywhere in your body, but you experience it as being centered in your brain, in the sixth and seventh chakras. You subjectively experience all the other chakras as "below you" in the spine. Any time you concentrate your mind on a chakra or draw energy down sushumna, you are moving Shiva-prana.

Shakti-prana. You subjectively experience surges of Shakti-prana as surges of strength, desire, and emotion "rising up" within you. Shakti-prana is everywhere but is most active in the coccyx and sacrum: the first and second chakras. Any time you draw energy up your spine, you are raising Shakti-prana.

Uniting Shiva-prana and Shakti-prana. Dr. Motoyama taught that Shiva-prana and Shakti-prana must reunite inside each chakra. This will purify and awaken each chakra. In practice this means you must learn to draw your energies into the chakras and concentrate your mind on them.

Pranayama and mantras. Although you are unaware of it, during every inhalation a little Shiva-prana is drawn into your body and down sushumna, and a little Shakti-prana is drawn up sushumna. You can influence the movements of these pranas by using mantras and visualizations during pranayama.

Before illustrating specific pranayama techniques, I will describe the "SoHam" and "HamSah" mantras. These mantras are commonly used when practicing pranayama. They deepen your awareness of how thought, breath, and prana are interrelated.

SoHam. The sanskrit "sah" rhymes with the english "saw." The sanskrit "aham" rhymes with the english "the-thumb." When sah and aham are blended into a single word, the sanskrit pronunciation changes to So-Ham, which rhymes with "toe-thumb."

The sanskrit word "sah" means "that." "That" refers to "The Source of All Things." The sanskrit "aham" means "I." SoHam means "That I Am."

HamSah. The syllables of the SoHam mantra can be reversed and mentally chanted as HamSo. But when chanted in this sequence the syllable "So" returns to its original pronunciation as "Sah." HamSo becomes HamSah. Ham-Sah rhymes with "thumb-saw."

HamSah means "I Am That."

SoHam emphasizes Shiva-prana, a sense of expanding, a sense of accepting.

HamSah emphasizes Shakti-prana, a sense of tensing, a sense of yearning.

Yang pranayama. There are four phases of controlled breathing: inhalation, retention, exhalation, and the pause after exhalation. Yang pranayama focuses on the rhythm of inhalation-retention-exhalation. Yin pranayama focuses on the pause after exhalation.

Yang pranayama is used to increase the flow of Shiva-prana and Shakti-prana within sushumna.

Patanjali does not use the terms yang or yin, but his description of pranayama falls neatly into these categories. What I refer to as yang pranayama is defined by Patanjali as controlling the rhythm of inhalation-retention-exhalation. Patanjali is not specific about what these rhythms should be because different yoginis use a variety of pranayama techniques and rhythms. (Patanjali 2.49-2.50)

Rhythms of yang pranayama. Dr. Motoyama taught that there is no rhythm of pranayama that works best for everyone, so he encouraged yoginis to experiment. My colleagues have reported several effective rhythms of inhalation-retention-exhalation. These include 4-8-4 and 4-16-4 and 8-4-8 and 8-8-8. Each count is about one second of time. When learning pranayama, you might mentally count these numbers, but in time, counting becomes unnecessary.

I suggest that you don't count when learning pran-ayama, at least not in the beginning. Just inhale for a comfortable length of time, hold your breath for a comfortable length of time, and then exhale for a comfortable length of time. After you are established in a comfortable rhythm, you might mentally count the seconds of each stage of your breathing. This will give you an idea of what kind of rhythm works for you, but counting is not essential. What is essential is a calm, consistent rhythm of breathing.

Whatever your rhythm of inhalation-retention-exhalation, each complete breath cycle should last 16-24 seconds or longer, depending on how calm you become.

SoHam yang pranayama. Although Shiva-prana and Shakti-prana are both affected by pranayama, it is possible to emphasize one over the other. This technique emphasizes drawing Shiva-prana down sushumna and into a chakra.

I have used the first chakra as an illustration of this technique because when you learn to draw Shiva-prana all the way down to the first chakra, you will be able to draw Shiva-prana down into any of the other chakras.

1. *Begin* by sitting calmly with an upright spine for five minutes. It is helpful to imagine sushumna as a column of light that starts at your coccyx, runs up your spine, and exits through Brahman's Gate at the top of your head.

2. *Inhale* while mentally chanting a long "SOOO." Imagine Shiva-prana flowing down sushumna and into the first chakra.

3. *Hold* the Shiva-prana in your first chakra while holding your breath for as long as you feel comfortable. While holding your breath, keep your glottis, your throat, open. This helps prevent the buildup of pressure in your head.

4. *Exhale* while mentally chanting a long "HAMMM." Imagine the Shiva-prana flowing up sushumna and out Brahman's Gate at the top of your head.

5. *Now begin again* with the next inhalation.

Learning the technique.
It will probably take some time to become comfortable with this pranayama technique. I suggest that you practice every day for a couple of weeks. Try to complete 7 or 14 or 21 breaths, without pause and without strain.

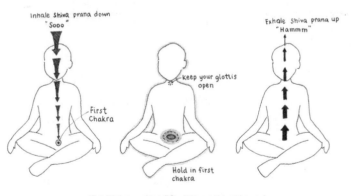

SOHAM YANG PRANAYAMA

HamSah yang pranayama. Although Shiva-prana and Shakti-prana are both affected by pranayama, it is possible to emphasize one over the other. This technique emphasizes drawing Shakti-prana up sushumna and into a chakra.

I have used the seventh chakra as an illustration of this technique because when you learn to draw Shakti-prana all the way up to Brahman's Gate, you will be able to draw Shakti-prana up into any of the other chakras.

1. *Begin* by sitting calmly with an upright spine for five minutes. It is helpful to imagine sushumna as a column of light that starts at your coccyx, runs up your spine, and exits through Brahman's Gate at the top of your head.

2. *Inhale* while mentally chanting a long "HAMMM." Imagine Shakti-prana rising from the first chakra, up sushumna, piercing Brahman's Gate, and rising above your head.

3. *Hold* the Shakti-prana above your head while holding your breath for as long as you feel comfortable. While holding your breath, keep your glottis, your throat, open. This helps prevent the buildup of pressure in your head.

4. *Exhale* while mentally chanting a long "SAHHH." Imagine the Shakti-prana descending through Brahman's Gate, and continuing all the way down sushumna to your first chakra.

5. *Now begin again* with the next inhalation.

Learning the technique.
It will probably take some time to become comfortable with this pranayama technique. I suggest that you practice every day for a couple of weeks. Try to complete 7 or 14 or 21 breaths, without pause and without strain.

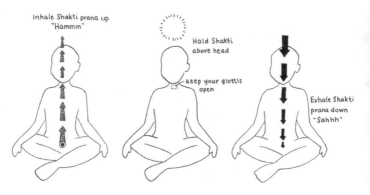

Inhale Shakti prana up
"Hammm"

Hold Shakti
above head

keep your glottis
open

Exhale Shakti
prana down
"Sahhh"

HAMSAH YANG PRANAYAMA

Yin pranayama. Let us recall the four phases of breathing: inhalation, retention, exhalation, and the pause after exhalation. Yang pranayama focuses on the rhythm of inhalation-retention-exhalation. Yin pranayama focuses on the pause after exhalation.

Yin pranayama focuses on the breathless pause that occurs after an unforced exhalation. In this phase of the breathing cycle, the ribcage is neither expanded nor contracted, and the diaphragm is completely relaxed. The effortless extension of this breathless pause is yin pranayama.

What I refer to as yin pranayama, Patanjali calls "the fourth pranayama." Patanjali writes that this pranayama is the "withdrawal of inhalation and exhalation" or "transcends inhalation and exhalation." Inhalation and exhalation are automatically reduced as the breathless pause extends. The breathing of master yogis is so small as to be undetectable. In this sense, the inhalation and exhalation have been transcended. (Patanjali 2.51)

Breathless pause. The breathless pause of yin pran-ayama does not extend with muscular effort; it only extends if you become physically, energetically, emo-tionally, and mentally quiet.

When practicing yin pranayama, pay close attention to the breathless, peaceful pause after each exhalation. As you become calm, it will become clear that every vritti in your chitta — every sensation, emotion, and thought — affects this breathless state. Some vrit-tis, such as feelings of peace, take you deeper into the breathless state; other vrittis, such as disturbing memories, arouse your breath and break the calm. Extending the breathless state and controlling the vrittis in your chitta are two sides of the same coin. Longer and longer periods of the breathless state are the physical signs of the purification of your chitta.

SoHam yin pranayama. This form of yin pranayama emphasizes relaxing and opening to Shiva-prana.

1. Concentrate on a chakra.

2. When an inhalation arises, mentally chant a brief, gentle "SO."

3. When the exhalation falls out, mentally chant a brief, gentle "HAM."

4. Enjoy the breathless calm while focused on the chakra, and wait for the next inhalation to arise.

5. As your breathing becomes more shallow and less frequent, and the breathless pauses become longer, you may start to feel energy movement, or see astral lights, or hear nada sounds. Try to become absorbed into these internal phenomena. If an afflicted or a nonafflicted vritti arises, then deal with it appropriately.

6. Continue for as long as you wish.

HamSah yin pranayama. This form of yin pranayama emphasizes awakening and raising Shakti-prana.

1. Concentrate on a chakra.

2. When an inhalation arises, mentally chant a brief, gentle "HAM."

3. When the exhalation falls out, mentally chant a brief, gentle "SAH."

4. Enjoy the breathless calm while focused on the chakra, and wait for the next inhalation to arise.

5. As your breathing becomes more shallow and less frequent, and the breathless pauses become longer, you may start to feel energy movement, or see astral lights, or hear nada sounds. Try to become absorbed into these internal phenomena. If an afflicted or a nonafflicted vritti arises, then deal with it appropriately.

6. Continue for as long as you wish.

Pratyahara. Pratyahara is the fifth limb of yogic control. Pratyhara is the conscious withdrawal of energy from the sensory nerves. You are endowed with an unconscious, instinctive ability to withdraw energy from the sensory nerves so you can sleep. Pratyahara is the conscious cultivation of this instinctive ability. Patanjali defines pratyahara as "the withdrawal of the senses from their objects as the mind withdraws into its own nature." (Patanjali 1.10, 2.54-2.55)

Patanjali defines sleep as "the desire to be absent" from the present state of consciousness. It is the desire to be absent that makes us "sleepy" when we are bored. Sleep is an unconscious state of sensory withdrawal, but a yogini wants to develop a conscious state of sensory withdrawal. The pratyahara of a yogini does not result in unconscious sleep but in conscious awareness of astral and causal phenomena.

A master of pratyahara is difficult to disturb in her meditation because the energy in her nerves is withdrawn. Sheltered in a self-created cave of sensory silence, her meditation is undisturbed by the endless prickings of the senses and the mental responses they arouse.

Pratyahara is developed by a long and sustained practice of pranayama, or meditating on the nada sounds, or meditating on the heart chakra. (Patanjali 1.23-1.29, 2.49-2.55, 3.34)

Dharana. Dharana is the sixth limb of yogic control. Dharana is usually translated as "concentration." Patanjali defines it as "binding the mind to one place." Focusing on the physical location of a chakra is dharana. (Patanjali 3.1)

The distinguishing aspect of dharana is that it requires willpower and imagination to create a focus for your awareness. For example, when you try to concentrate on your second chakra, you start by imagining it somewhere in your sacrum or lower abdomen. You try to feel how that area is affected by your breath, but you don't know for certain if you are feeling the chakra or just a muscle or an organ. You might find it difficult to discriminate internal perceptions from wishful imaginings. Nonetheless, your effort to concentrate gradually calms your mind and gathers your Shiva-prana and Shakti-prana into the chakra.

Dhyana. Dhyana is the seventh limb of yogic control. Dhyana is usually translated as "meditation." Patanjali defines it as "the extension of a single intention." Dhyana is your fascinated absorption with internal phenomena that arise as a result of your dharana. (Patanjali 3.2)

The distinguishing aspect of dhyana is that your focus is on something discovered within you, not something you have willfully imagined. For example, while holding your awareness on the physical location of a chakra, you might become aware of heat or pressure in that area, or astral lights at your third eye, or nada sounds ringing in your right ear. These phenomena are not created by your imagination. They are discovered by you. Your fascinated absorption into these phenomena is dhyana.

Samadhi. Samadhi is the eighth limb of yogic control. Samadhi is the highest state of meditative absorption. Patanjali defines it "as if empty of your own nature, the object of meditation alone shines forth." (Patanjali 3.3)

When practicing dharana and dhyana on a chakra, a yogini is relying on the energy she feels, the light she sees, or the sound she hears. Relying on these sensory impressions, even subtle sensory impressions, is not the same as identifying with a chakra. When a yogini so strongly identifies with the object of her meditation that her individual nature seems to become "shunya," empty, void, then she has entered into samadhi.

When a yogini enters into samadhi, she experiences a state of consciousness that includes both the object of her meditation and her meditating ego as parts of a greater whole. The philosophical question now becomes, "If I am able to see my ego as only a part of myself, then what am I?" The first and obvious answer is that you are not the ego you thought you were. The yogic answer is that your consciousness has been lifted to a higher level of astral or causal embodiment. You are now identifying with this larger embodiment and viewing your previous limited embodiment floating inside you. All forms of embodiment, great or small, are forms of ego. (Patanjali 3.38, 3.43)

More than empty. Describing samadhi as becoming empty or void does not do it justice. Simultaneous with the voiding of the ego is an expansion of the sense of Self and an intensification of feeling, of love, and of wisdom. This new sense of Self may not yet be the true Self, Purusha, but it is still an important stage of spiritual development.

Cosmic consciousness. The following is a description of a samadhi experienced in 1873 by Richard Maurice Bucke, a Canadian psychologist. The description is taken from his book "Cosmic Consciousness" in which he writes of his experience in the third person. His samadhi occurred unexpectedly, after a night of reading spiritual poetry with some friends.

"Directly afterwards came upon him a sense of exultation, of immense joyousness accompanied or immediately followed by an intellectual illumination quite impossible to describe. Into his brain streamed one momentary lightning-flash of the Brahmic Splendor which has ever since lightened his life; upon his heart fell one drop of Brahmic Bliss, leaving thenceforward for always an aftertaste of heaven. Among other things he did not come to believe, he saw and knew that the Cosmos is not dead matter but a living Presence, that the soul of man is immortal, that the universe is so built and ordered that without any peradventure all things work together for the good of each and all, that the foundation principle of the world is what we call love and that the happiness of everyone is in the long run absolutely certain."

Many stages of samadhi. Yoga teaches that there is not just one false ego but at least three: a physical ego, an astral ego, and a causal ego. A yogini must experience many stages of samadhi before she can discriminate the differences between her Purusha and the physical, astral, and causal bodies that ensheath her. Each new level of samadhi is more profound than the previous one. But she must not be seduced by the mystical powers she inherits in these new levels of existence. She must not be content to replace her previous physical identification with an astral or a causal one. She must not stop until she realizes the highest Purusha. (Patanjali 1.41-1.51, 2.16-2.27, 3.35-3.55, 4.34)

Centuries of Meditations. The following two quotations were written by Thomas Traherne, a 17th century English clergyman and mystic. They are meditations 1.29 and 1.30 of his "Centuries of Meditations."

"You never enjoy the world aright, till the Sea itself floweth in your veins, till you are clothed with the heavens, and crowned with the stars: and perceive yourself to be the sole heir of the whole world, and more than so, because men are in it who are every one sole heirs as well as you. Till you can sing and rejoice and delight in God, as misers do in gold, and Kings in sceptres, you never enjoy the world.

Till your spirit filleth the whole world, and the stars are your jewels; till you are as familiar with the ways of God in all Ages as with your walk and table: till you are intimately acquainted with that shady nothing out of which the world was made: till you love men so as to desire their happiness, with a thirst equal to the zeal of your own: till you delight in God for being good to all: you never enjoy the world…"

All you need is Love. One of our most prized possessions is a Japanese calligraphy by Dr. Motoyama. It translates as "God is Love."

In 1894 the great yogi Swami Sri Yukteswar wrote a treatise titled "The Holy Science." This brief but powerful collection of 84 sutras expresses the essence of yoga practice. In this book, Sri Yukteswar writes that the heart's natural love is the principal requisite to attain a holy life, that the true conception of a thing is only possible if it is felt by the heart, and only by feeling things with the heart is it possible to enter into samadhi with them. (Yukteswar 3.6, 3.19-3.20)

In his conclusion, Sri Yukteswar proclaims that the phrase "Love is God" is not just a sentimental poetic expression but is an aphorism of eternal truth. And he quotes approvingly from "The Lay of the Last Minstrel" by Sir Walter Scott:

> "Love rules the court, the camp, the grove,
> And men below, and saints above:
> For love is heaven and heaven is love."

Part 4.
Meditation.

Shiva and Shakti. The Unmanifest Absolute, God, Parabrahman manifests itself as a Duality of Powers. This Duality creates and sustains the worlds. One aspect of this duality is Shakti. Shakti is Creative Force. Shakti creates, sustains, and eventually dissolves all things. The other aspect of this duality is Shiva. Shiva is Consciousness or Feeling. Shiva gives Feeling and Consciousness to all things.

Reunification. The microcosmic reflections of these macrocosmic powers are called Shakti-prana and Shiva-prana. Your ability to visualize a chakra and hold your awareness on it is the power of intention, the power of your Shiva-prana. The energy that created your body, that you feel moving inside you is your Shakti-prana. The path of chakra meditation is to reunite these energies inside each of the chakras. This reunification first occurs in the physical dimension, then the astral, and then the causal. At each stage of reunification, the yogini experiences a form of samadhi.

Purification. When focusing your Shiva-prana and Shakti-prana into a chakra, it is inevitable that the vasanas and samskaras lying dormant within the chakra will become active vrittis. Effectively dealing with these vrittis is the process of chakra purification. But purifying the chakras is not a goal in itself. It is only a necessary step toward abandoning your false sense of self, the false conviction that you are your embodied forms.

Surrender. Dr. Motoyama said that you cannot crack the shell of your ego unless you surrender to something larger than yourself. He suggested that you use the last minutes of your meditations to surrender all your efforts to God, or Buddha, or any form of divinity that inspires you. Patanjali wrote that perfection in samadhi arises from dedication to Ishvara, the highest Purusha. The spiritual path is a deeply personal, deeply mystical blend of self-effort and self-surrender that each yogini must discover for herself. (Patanjali 1.23-1.28, 2.45)

Nyasa. Circulating your energy and awareness through all of the chakras is called "nyasa." Nyasa means to deliberately put something in a place. Nyasa can refer to carefully placing objects on an altar during religious rituals. The altar for a yogini is her spine, and the objects she places on it are her awareness and her energy: her Shiva-prana and her Shakti-prana. Working your way down the chakras is "descending nyasa." Working your way up the chakras is "ascending nyasa." One descending and one ascending nyasa is a complete cycle of nyasa.

PART 4. MEDITATION.

The various seeds of your karma, your desires and habits, are stored in different chakras, and they unfold at different times. This means that your chakras are varying in their degree of activity and dominance relative to each other. One of the fundamentally important things a yogini should try to do is balance the flow of energy moving through sushumna and the chakras. This makes it much easier to enter deeper meditative states. Nyasa is an effective way to do this.

Yang nyasa. There are several forms of nyasa. Outlined below is a nyasa that incorporates yang pranayama. If you practice one yang breath per chakra, it is a one-breath nyasa. If you practice two breaths per chakra, it is a two-breath nyasa. Three breaths per chakra is a three-breath nyasa, and so on. I have illustrated this technique with a one-breath nyasa.

Yang nyasa routine.
Begin by sitting calmly with an upright spine for five minutes. It is helpful to imagine sushumna as a column of light that starts at your coccyx, runs up your spine, and exits through Brahman's Gate at the top of your head.

Begin descending nyasa...
1. *Concentrate* on the seventh chakra and practice SoHam yang pranayama one time.
2. *Repeat* this for the sixth, fifth, fourth, third, second, and first chakras.
3. *Meditate* on the rebound. Feel all of sushumna. Become absorbed into the nada you hear, the light you see, or the energy you feel in sushumna. If an afflicted or a nonafflicted vritti arises, then deal with it appropriately.

Begin ascending nyasa…

1. *Concentrate* on the first chakra and practice HamSah yang pranayama one time.

2. *Repeat* this for the second, third, fourth, fifth, sixth, and seventh chakras.

3. *Meditate* on the rebound. Feel all of sushumna. Become absorbed into the nada you hear, the light you see, or the energy you feel in sushumna. If an afflicted or a nonafflicted vritti arises, then deal with it appropriately.

Length of practice. At a rate of one breath per chakra, it should take between 15 and 25 minutes for you to finish a complete cycle of yang nyasa. The exact amount of time depends on how long you meditate on the rebounds. If you wish to sit longer, then practice a two-breath or a three-breath nyasa.

Yin nyasa. Outlined below is a nyasa that incorporates yin pranayama. If you practice one yin breath per chakra, it is a one-breath nyasa. If you practice two breaths per chakra, it is a two-breath nyasa. Three breaths per chakra is a three-breath nyasa, and so on. I have illustrated this technique with a three-breath nyasa.

Yin nyasa routine.
Begin by sitting calmly with an upright spine for five minutes. It is helpful to imagine sushumna as a column of light that starts at your coccyx, runs up your spine, and exits through Brahman's Gate at the top of your head.

Begin descending nyasa…

1. *Concentrate* on the seventh chakra and practice SoHam yin pranayama for three breaths.
2. *Repeat* this for the sixth, fifth, fourth, third, second, and first chakras.
3. *Meditate* on the rebound. Feel all of sushumna. Become absorbed into the nada you hear, the light you see, or the energy you feel in sushumna. If an afflicted or a nonafflicted vritti arises, then deal with it appropriately.

Begin ascending nyasa…

1. *Concentrate* on the first chakra and practice HamSah yin pranayama for three breaths.

2. *Repeat* this for the second, third, fourth, fifth, sixth, and seventh chakras.

3. *Meditate* on the rebound. Feel all of sushumna. Become absorbed into the nada you hear, the light you see, or the energy you feel in sushumna. If an afflicted or a nonafflicted vritti arises, then deal with it appropriately.

Length of practice. At a rate of three breaths per chakra, it should take between 15 and 25 minutes for you to finish a complete cycle of yin nyasa. The exact amount of time depends on how long you meditate on the rebounds. It is an easy matter to shorten or lengthen the time of a nyasa practice by decreasing or increasing the number of breaths per chakra.

Bija mantras. There is a form of nyasa that is not co-ordinated with your breathing. It is practiced while mentally chanting bija mantras. "Bija" means seed. Bija mantras are the "seed sounds" of the chakras. Mentally chanting these mantras stimulates the chakras and makes it easier to feel and concentrate on them. The bija mantra for each chakra is listed below.

Sahasrara	OM	*Rhymes with home*
Ajna	OM	*Rhymes with home*
Vishuddha	HAM	*Rhymes with thumb*
Anahata	YAM	*Rhymes with thumb*
Manipura	RAM	*Rhymes with thumb*
Svadhisthana	VAM	*Rhymes with thumb*
Muladhara	LAM	*Rhymes with thumb*

An alternative pronunciation ends each bija mantra with an "ng" sound like "tongue" rather than an "mmm" sound like "thumb." This alternative pronunciation subtly restricts the flow of breath. Some students find it more effective. Others find it too aggressive.

Sahasrara	OHNG	*Oh ending with "ng," like tongue*
Ajna	OHNG	*Oh ending with "ng," like tongue*
Vishuddha	HUNG	*Rhymes with tongue*
Anahata	YUNG	*Rhymes with tongue*
Manipura	RUNG	*Rhymes with tongue*
Svadhisthana	VUNG	*Rhymes with tongue*
Muladhara	LUNG	*Rhymes with tongue*

Bija mantra chanting. The basic technique of bija mantra meditation is quite simple:

1. *Concentrate* on a chakra.

2. *Mentally chant* its bija mantra.

3. *Meditate* on the rebound.

4. *Repeat* as many times as you wish.

Rhythm of chanting. Some yoginis chant the bija just once and then meditate on the rebound. Others chant the bija three or four times and then meditate on the rebound.

Some yoginis meditate on the rebound a long time before chanting again: this is a slow rhythm. Others meditate on the rebound for just a few seconds before chanting again: this is a fast rhythm.

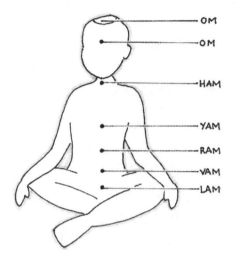

OM
OM
HAM
YAM
RAM
VAM
LAM

BIJA MANTRAS

Bija nyasa. Begin by sitting calmly with an upright spine for five minutes. It is helpful to imagine sushumna as a column of light that starts at your coccyx, runs up your spine, and exits through Brahman's Gate at the top of your head.

Begin descending nyasa…

1. *Bring* your awareness to the seventh chakra and mentally chant "OM."

2. *Move* your awareness to the sixth chakra and mentally chant "OM."

3. *Move* your awareness to the fifth chakra and mentally chant "HAM."

4. *Move* your awareness to the fourth chakra and mentally chant "YAM."

5. *Move* your awareness to the third chakra and mentally chant "RAM."

6. *Move* your awareness to the second chakra and mentally chant "VAM."

7. *Move* your awareness to the first chakra and mentally chant "LAM."

8. *Meditate on the rebound.* Feel all of sushumna. Become absorbed into the nada you hear, the light you see, or the energy you feel. If an afflicted or a nonafflicted vritti arises, then deal with it appropriately.

Begin ascending nyasa…

1. *Bring* your awareness to the first chakra and mentally chant "LAM."

2. *Move* your awareness to the second chakra and mentally chant "VAM."

3. *Move* your awareness to the third chakra and mentally chant "RAM."

4. *Move* your awareness to the fourth chakra and mentally chant "YAM."

5. *Move* your awareness to the fifth chakra and mentally chant "HAM."

6. *Move* your awareness to the sixth chakra and mentally chant "OM."

7. *Move* your awareness to the seventh chakra and mentally chant "OM."

8. *Meditate on the rebound.* Feel all of sushumna. Become absorbed into the nada you hear, the light you see, or the energy you feel. If an afflicted or a nonafflicted vritti arises, then deal with it appropriately.

Length of practice. Bija nyasa is the most variable of nyasa practices. Depending on how many times you chant and how long you meditate on each rebound, it can take anywhere from 3 to 30 minutes to finish a complete cycle of bija nyasa. I suggest you that you start with a rhythm of one minute per chakra.

Three-week cycle of nyasa meditation. Ancient yoga handbooks were written for people who did not lead a householder's life or have family responsibilites. These yogis were able to practice three or four times per day. Although admirable, such a schedule is not realistic in the modern world. Assuming that a beginning meditator will sit three or four times per week, I suggest the following three-week program.

Week 1:
Yang nyasa.

Week 2:
Yin nyasa.

Week 3:
Bija nyasa.

Now start the cycle over again, beginning with yang nyasa.

In one year's time, you will have gone through this three-week cycle 17 times. This should be enough repetition for you to assess the effects of the three different nyasa techniques. As you move into your second year, I suggest that you let go of the rigid three-week cycle and practice whichever form of nyasa you think would be most effective for you on any given day.

Meditating on one chakra. Dr. Motoyama said, "The same practices that are of great benefit at one stage of your spiritual growth can become a great hindrance at a different stage." No routine or technique will always be effective because your physical energies, astral emotions, and causal thoughts are constantly changing.

I believe nyasa practice is the fundamentally important technique, but even it will not always be the most effective practice for everyone, or for every meditation session. Sometimes it is best to focus on just one chakra.

After you have become familiar with the various forms of nyasa, I suggest that you systematically focus on one chakra per week for seven weeks. Keep a record of your experiences, and if you find one chakra generates particularly useful results, then focus on it for a few weeks and then reassess. I encourage you to return to nyasa practice whenever you feel the need. Dr. Motoyama cautioned against the overuse or overdevelopment of any one chakra.

Bija pranayama. This technique is an effective way to focus on one chakra. It is practiced by mentally chanting "OM" with the inhalation and a "bija" with the exhalation. It can be used with both yin and yang pranayamas.

For example, if you wish to focus on manipura, the third chakra, you might proceed as follows:

Begin by sitting calmly with an upright spine for five minutes. It is helpful to imagine sushumna as a column of light that starts at your coccyx, runs up your spine, and exits through Brahman's Gate at the top of your head.

1. *Concentrate* on the third chakra and practice yin pranayama. Mentally chant a brief, gentle "OM" with the inhalation, and a brief, gentle "RAM" with the exhalation. Practice for 10 or 15 minutes, or more.

2. *Transition* to yang pranayama. Mentally chant a long "OOOM" with the inhalation, hold your breath for as long as comfortable, and then mentally chant a long "RAMMM" with the exhalation. Practice 7, or 14, or 21 breaths.

3. *Meditate* on the rebound for ten minutes or more.

Little by little. The path of yoga means becoming less and less attached to the vrittis in your chitta, becoming less and less attached to who you think you are. As you draw away from who you think you are, you stop competing and comparing yourself with others. This gradually erodes vanity, envy, and jealousy. As you become more insightful into your own problems, you become more compassionate toward the problems of others; you become more patient, more calm, and more kind. These are spiritual treasures that accumulate almost imperceptibly, but they are of lasting value. Don't overlook them.

Beyond the chakras. Awakening the chakras is important, but it is not the final goal of spiritual life. Chakras are centers of consciousness and energy that create and maintain your three bodies as you work through your karma. But the spiritual path as outlined by Dr. Motoyama is to awaken to an existence that is beyond the three bodies, to an existence beyond karma and the chakras: this is the realm of Purusha. Even Purusha is not the highest goal. Beyond Purusha is the Absolute: "...that shady nothing out of which the world was made." (Traherne 1.30)

Further Resources

It is my hope that this book proves to be a practical guide to the theory and techniques of chakra meditation. I also hope it might be a bridge to deeper philosophical works. Listed below are the texts that I have found most useful in my own studies.

Aranya, Swami Hariharananda (2012) Yoga Philosophy of Patanjali with Bhasvati. 4th edition. University of Calcutta, Calcutta.

Bryant, Edwin F. (2009) The Yoga Sutras of Patanjali. North Point Press, New York, New York.

Chapple, Christopher (2008) Yoga and the Luminous. State University of New York, Albany, New York.

Motoyama, Dr. Hiroshi (2009) Being and the Logic of Interactive Function. Human Sciences Press, Tokyo, Japan.

Motoyama, Dr. Hiroshi (2006) Varieties of Mystical Experience. Human Sciences Press, Tokyo, Japan.

Motoyama, Dr. Hiroshi (2003) Awakening the Chakras and Emancipation. Human Sciences Press, Tokyo, Japan.

Traherne, Thomas (1958) Centuries, Poems, and Thanksgivings. Oxford University Press, London.

Yogananda, Paramahansa (1995) God Talks with Arjuna. Self-Realization Fellowship, Los Angeles, California.

Yogananda, Paramahansa (1982) The Science of Religion. Self-Realization Fellowship, Los Angeles, California.

Yukteswar, Swami Sri (1977) The Holy Science. Self-Realization Fellowship, Los Angeles, California.

Subject Index

About the author

Paul Grilley was born in Seattle, Washington, in 1958. He has practiced yoga since reading "The Autobiography of a Yogi" in the summer of 1979.

He lived and taught yoga classes in Los Angeles from 1982 until 1994. He also took classes in kinesiology at UCLA.

Paul and his wife, Suzee became students of Dr. Hiroshi Motoyama in 1990.

Paul and Suzee moved to Ashland, Oregon in 1994, where they still have a home. In 2000 he earned a Master's Degree from St. John's College, Santa Fe, and in 2005 he was awarded an Honorary Ph.D. from the California Institute for Human Science. The Ph.D. was in recognition of his book and DVDs promoting the practice and theory of yin yoga.